KETO FOOD CHOICES FOR PEDIATRIC DRUG RESISTANT EPILEPSY

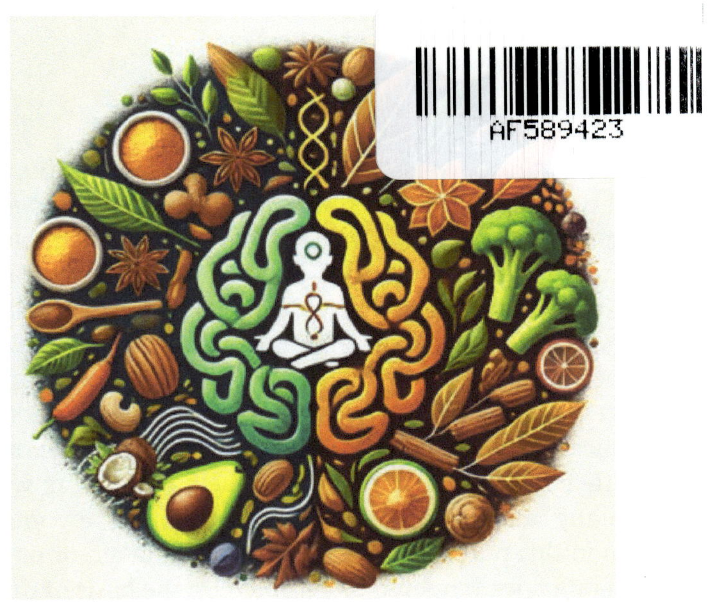

Dr. A.J. Hemamalini
Soma Basu

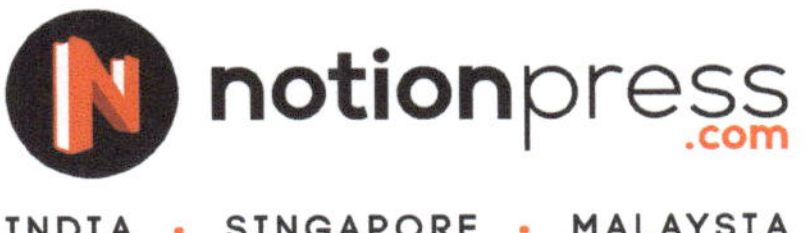

INDIA • SINGAPORE • MALAYSIA

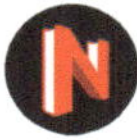

ISBN 979-8-89906-998-7

ABOUT THE BOOK

"Keto Food Choices for Pediatric Drug-Resistant Epilepsy" is a practical guide for families and caregivers seeking safe, effective dietary solutions beyond anti-seizure medications. This book simplifies the ketogenic diet, offering clear, Indian-cuisine-friendly options tailored to the unique needs of children with drug-resistant epilepsy. Packed with food lists, portion guides, and meal planning tips, it empowers readers to make informed choices, supporting seizure control through nutrition. Whether you're starting out or refining your keto journey, this essential companion helps you navigate every step with confidence.

FOREWORD

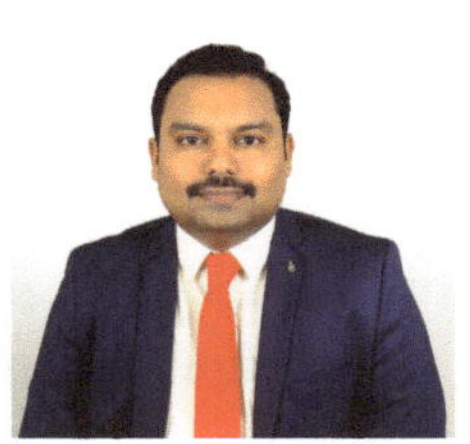

As a pediatric neurologist and epileptologist, I have walked alongside many families facing the formidable challenge of drug-resistant epilepsy. For these families, every seizure is not just a clinical event but an emotional upheaval—a reminder of the uncertainties that define their daily lives. When medications fall short, and seizures persist despite our best medical efforts, the search for alternative, effective treatments becomes urgent and deeply personal.

The ketogenic diet has stood the test of time as a proven therapy for drug-resistant epilepsy, offering significant seizure reduction and, in many cases, life-changing improvement. Yet, while its scientific foundation is robust, translating this therapy into practical, everyday food choices is often where families feel overwhelmed. This is especially true when navigating cultural dietary patterns, feeding young children, and maintaining nutritional balance alongside medical goals.

"***Keto Food Choices for Pediatric Drug-Resistant Epilepsy***" serves as an essential guide for this very journey. The author has skillfully bridged the gap between complex clinical guidance and accessible, family-friendly solutions. With an emphasis on culturally relevant options and clear, actionable recommendations, this book equips caregivers with the tools they need to confidently implement the ketogenic diet in their homes.

What makes this work especially commendable is its blend of scientific rigor and compassionate understanding. It recognizes that families are not just looking for recipes—they are searching for hope, reassurance, and a sustainable path forward. Through practical food lists, thoughtful meal ideas, and easy-to-understand explanations, this book brings clarity to what often feels like a daunting process.

I am confident that this resource will empower families and caregivers, helping them transform the ketogenic diet from a theoretical concept into a meaningful, effective strategy for seizure control. It stands as a testament to the shared commitment of healthcare providers, patients, and families working together toward brighter outcomes.

I wholeheartedly recommend this book to anyone involved in the care of a child with drug-resistant epilepsy. May it guide you, encourage you, and remind you that every step toward seizure freedom is a step worth taking.

Dr. Ranjith Kumar Manokaran

Associate Professor, Division of Pediatric Neurology and Epileptology

Senior Consultant Pediatric Neurologist & Epileptologist

Sri Ramachandra Institute of Higher Education and Research

Porur, Chennai, Tamil Nadu, India

PREFACE

Epilepsy has long challenged both patients and healthcare providers, especially when conventional treatments fall short. Drug-resistant epilepsy where seizures persist despite the use of two or more appropriate anti-seizure medications presents an especially difficult journey for families and clinicians alike. In these circumstances, dietary therapies such as the ketogenic diet offer a beacon of hope. This book, "***Keto Food Choices for Pediatric Drug-Resistant Epilepsy***," emerges from that hope, and from a deep commitment to supporting children and adults living with refractory seizures.

The ketogenic diet is not just a nutritional choice; it is a carefully balanced, therapeutic intervention that demands precision, dedication, and a clear understanding of food composition and metabolic needs. While its efficacy is well-documented in reducing seizure frequency and improving quality of life, many caregivers and families find themselves overwhelmed by the complexities of daily meal planning. Questions about suitable ingredients, cultural preferences, child-friendly meals, and nutritional adequacy are common, and deserve thoughtful, practical answers.

This book is designed to be that trusted companion. It bridges the gap between clinical recommendations and everyday practice, especially for families seeking keto-friendly food choices within familiar culinary traditions. The recipes, food lists, and guidelines provided here are tailored for drug-resistant epilepsy, keeping in mind the strict carbohydrate limits and the high-fat requirements of the diet.

Moreover, we have paid special attention to cultural diversity, ensuring the options are adaptable to various regional and personal tastes. Whether you are a parent seeking safe and tasty meal ideas for your child, or a healthcare provider looking to guide your patients, this book aims to equip you with clarity, confidence, and culinary inspiration.

As you explore these pages, remember that you are not alone on this journey. Behind every meal plan and recipe lies the shared determination of countless families and professionals working tirelessly to unlock better days, one meal at a time. We hope this book becomes a source of practical guidance and gentle encouragement, lighting the path toward improved seizure control and a better quality of life.

Dr. A.J. Hemamalini & Soma Basu

DISCLAIMER

The information and recipes provided in *Keto Food Choices for Pediatric Drug-Resistant Epilepsy* are intended solely for educational purposes and are designed with consideration for children between the age of 1 to 3 years. It is important to emphasize that the ketogenic diet for epilepsy is a therapeutic and highly individualized intervention—**one size does not fit all**.

Dietary requirements can vary greatly based on a child's age, gender, seizure type, seizure severity, reflux status, allergy profile, nutritional needs, and prescribed ketogenic ratio. Therefore, proper planning and individualized customization of the diet are essential. While the types of ingredients used in the recipes generally remain the same across ketogenic ratios (from 1:1 to 3:1), **the quantity of each ingredient is adjusted** based on the prescribed ratio for the individual child. Therefore, even though the recipe and ingredient list may appear similar, the proportions will vary according to the specific ketogenic ratio required.

Parents and caregivers are strongly advised to consult a pediatric neurologist / epileptologist and a certified ketogenic dietitian before initiating any of the recipes or dietary approaches outlined in this book. Similarly, healthcare professionals and dietitians are encouraged to collaborate with trained ketogenic dietician and pediatric epileptologists before recommending these recipes to patients.

The authors and publishers do not assume any responsibility or liability for any adverse effects resulting from the use of the information or recipes provided herein without appropriate medical supervision and individualized dietary management.

TABLE OF CONTENTS

INTRODUCTION

Drug Resistant Epilepsy

Epilepsy is a chronic neurological disorder characterized by the occurrence of recurrent, unprovoked seizures, resulting from abnormal, excessive neuronal activity in the brain. It affects individuals of all ages but is particularly significant in the pediatric population due to its impact on neurodevelopment. Despite the availability of a wide range of anti-seizure medications, approximately 20–30% of pediatric patients develop drug-resistant epilepsy (DRE), defined as the failure to achieve sustained seizure freedom after adequate trials of at least two appropriately chosen and tolerated anti-seizure medications. In such cases, alternative therapies, including dietary treatments, become essential. One of the most well-established dietary interventions for pediatric epilepsy is the ketogenic diet (KD), a high-fat, low-carbohydrate, and adequate-protein regimen designed to mimic the metabolic effects of fasting.

What does Ketogenic Diet Ratio mean?

The ketogenic diet typically utilizes specific fat-to-carbohydrate-plus-protein ratios, expressed as 1:1, 2:1, 3:1, or 4:1. These ratios reflect the grams of fat relative to the combined grams of carbohydrates and proteins; for example, a 1:1 ratio indicates that for every 1 grams of fat, there is a total of 1 gram of carbohydrates plus protein.

Parents or caregivers should not change the ketogenic diet ratio on their own when it's being used for epilepsy treatment. The ketogenic diet for epilepsy is a prescribed medical nutrition therapy, not just a low-carb lifestyle.

It's tailored to the child's age, weight, seizure type, medical history, lab values. Changing the ratio (e.g., from 1:1 to 2:1) can throw off the carefully balanced fat-to-carb/protein proportions needed to maintain ketosis which is the therapeutic state that helps control seizures.

Adjustments *can* be made, but only by a treating team, usually consisting of a pediatric neurologist /epileptologist or a certified ketogenic dietitian.

Mechanism of action of Ketogenic Diet is Drug Resistant Epilepsy

Under a regular diet, which is typically rich in carbohydrates, the body primarily uses glucose as its main source of energy. Carbohydrates are broken down into glucose, which enters cells through insulin-mediated pathways and fuels brain activity. In individuals with epilepsy, this glucose-driven metabolism may support higher neuronal excitability, contributing to the generation of seizures in some cases.

In contrast, the ketogenic diet (KD) dramatically reduces carbohydrate intake and provides high amounts of fat with adequate protein. As a result, the body shifts from glucose metabolism to fat metabolism, entering a state known as **nutritional ketosis.** In ketosis, the liver breaks down fatty acids into **ketone bodies**—mainly **beta-hydroxybutyrate (BHB)**, **acetoacetate**, and **acetone**—which serve as alternative energy substrates for the brain.

Several mechanisms by which the ketogenic diet contributes to seizure control include:

1. **Altered Energy Metabolism**: Ketone bodies provide a more efficient and stable source of energy than glucose, enhancing mitochondrial function and ATP production. Improved mitochondrial health reduces neuronal hyperexcitability and protects against seizure generation.

2. **Neurotransmitter Balance**: The KD increases the synthesis and release of **GABA** (gamma-aminobutyric acid), the brain's major inhibitory neurotransmitter, while reducing levels of **glutamate**, the primary excitatory neurotransmitter. This shift toward inhibitory signaling dampens excessive neuronal firing.
3. **Reduced Oxidative Stress**: Ketogenic metabolism reduces the production of reactive oxygen species (ROS) and enhances antioxidant defenses, protecting neurons from oxidative damage, which is often linked to seizure activity.
4. **Ion Channel Modulation**: The KD influences the function of potassium and calcium ion channels, stabilizing neuronal membranes and reducing hyperexcitability.
5. **mTOR Pathway Inhibition**: The mammalian target of rapamycin (mTOR) signaling pathway, involved in cell growth and excitability, is downregulated by the KD. mTOR inhibition has been associated with reduced epileptogenesis in experimental models.
6. **Gut Microbiome Changes**: Emerging evidence suggests that the KD alters the composition of the gut microbiota, leading to production of metabolites that may have anticonvulsant effects.

Thus, compared to a high carbohydrate diet, the ketogenic diet induces a fundamental shift in brain metabolism and neurotransmission that collectively stabilizes neuronal activity and reduces the likelihood of seizures.

1:1 RATIO KETO RECIPES

BANANA MILKSHAKE

Nutritive Value

Nutrient	Value
Energy (kcal)	158.47
Carbohydrates (g)	9.11
Protein (g)	3.08
Fat (g)	12.19

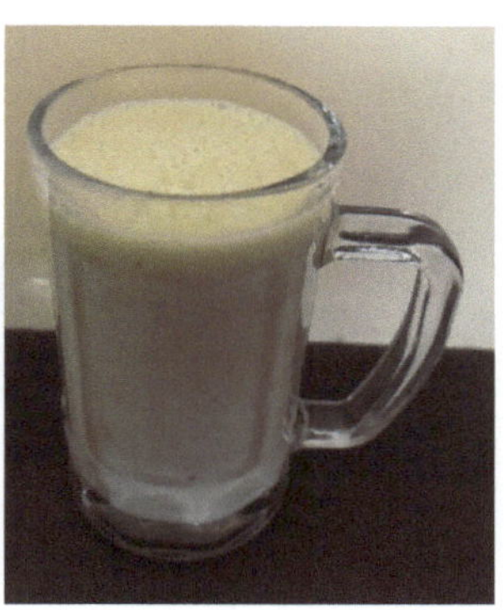

128 ml

List of Ingredients

Ingredients	Quantity
Banana	39 g
Soya Milk Unsweetened	78 ml
Coconut Oil	11 ml

Method

- Chop 39g banana into small pieces.
- Blend with 78ml unsweetened soya milk.
- Add 11ml coconut oil.
- Blend until smooth and creamy.
- Serve it.

Recipe by – Soma Basu

APPLE MILKSHAKE

Nutritive Value

Nutrient	Value
Energy (kcal)	158.47
Carbohydrates (g)	9.11
Protein (g)	3.08
Fat (g)	12.19

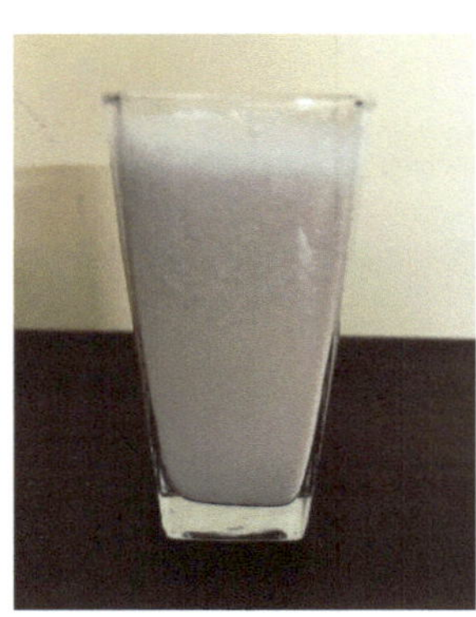

177 ml

List of Ingredients

Ingredients	Quantity
Apple	70 g
Soya Milk Unsweetened	96 ml
Coconut Oil	11 ml

Method

- Chop 70g apple into small pieces.
- Blend with 96ml unsweetened soya milk.
- Add 11ml coconut oil.
- Blend until smooth and creamy.
- Serve it.

Recipe by – Soma Basu

SAPOTA MILKSHAKE

Nutritive Value

Nutrient	Value
Energy (kcal)	158.47
Carbohydrates (g)	9.11
Protein (g)	3.08
Fat (g)	12.19

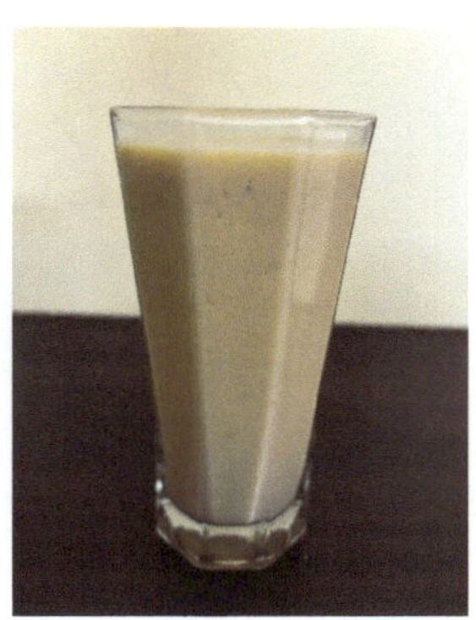

153 ml

List of Ingredients

Ingredients	Quantity
Sapota	66 g
Soya Milk Unsweetened	77 ml
Coconut Oil	10 ml

Method

- Chop 66g sapota into small pieces.
- Blend with 77ml unsweetened soya milk.
- Add 10ml coconut oil.
- Blend until smooth and creamy.
- Serve it.

Recipe by – Soma Basu

POMEGRANATE MILKSHAKE

Nutritive Value

Nutrient	Value
Energy (kcal)	158.47
Carbohydrates (g)	9.11
Protein (g)	3.08
Fat (g)	12.19

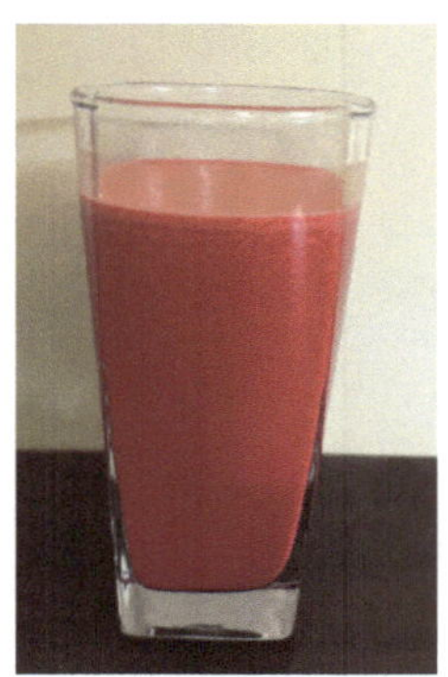

153 ml

List of Ingredients

Ingredients	Quantity
Pomegranate	79 g
Soya Milk Unsweetened	63 ml
Coconut Oil	11 ml

Method

- Chop 79g pomegranate into small pieces.
- Blend with 63ml unsweetened soya milk.
- Add 11ml coconut oil.
- Blend until smooth and creamy.
- Serve it.

Recipe by – Soma Basu

PAPAYA MILKSHAKE

Nutritive Value

Nutrient	Value
Energy (kcal)	158.47
Carbohydrates (g)	9.11
Protein (g)	3.08
Fat (g)	12.19

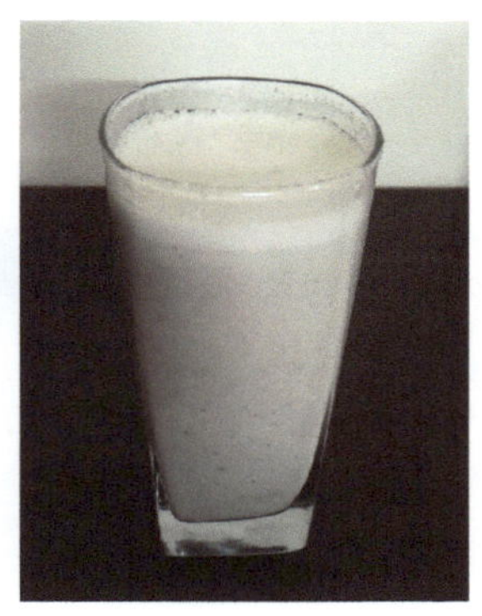

305 ml

List of Ingredients

Ingredients	Quantity
Papaya	198 g
Soya Milk Unsweetened	96 ml
Coconut Oil	11 ml

Method

- Chop 198g papaya into small pieces.
- Blend with 96ml unsweetened soya milk.
- Add 11ml coconut oil.
- Blend until smooth and creamy.
- Serve it.

Recipe by – Soma Basu

CARROT MILKSHAKE

Nutritive Value

Nutrient	Value
Energy (kcal)	158.47
Carbohydrates (g)	9.11
Protein (g)	3.08
Fat (g)	12.19

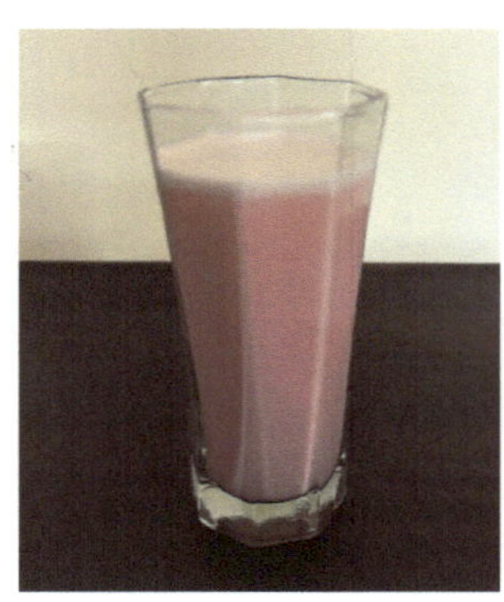

322 ml

List of Ingredients

Ingredients	Quantity
Carrot	164 g
Soya Milk Unsweetened	47 ml
Almond Milk Unsweetened	100 ml
Coconut Oil	11 ml

Method

- Chop 164g carrot into small pieces.
- Blend with 47ml unsweetened soya milk and 100 ml almond milk.
- Add 11ml coconut oil.
- Blend until smooth and creamy.
- Serve it.

Recipe by – Soma Basu

BEETROOT MILKSHAKE

Nutritive Value

Nutrient	Value
Energy (kcal)	158.47
Carbohydrates (g)	9.11
Protein (g)	3.08
Fat (g)	12.19

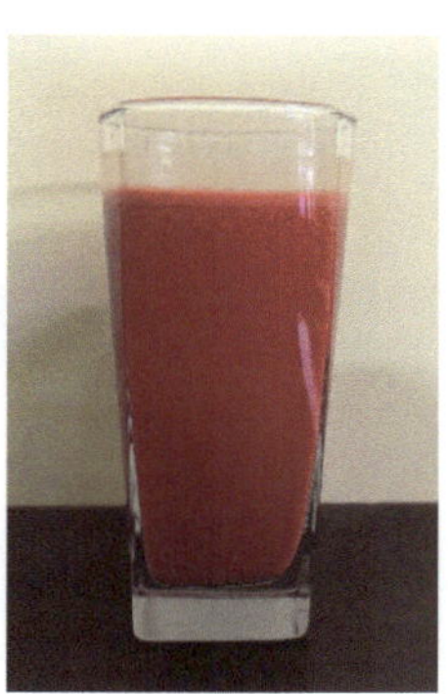

316 ml

List of Ingredients

Ingredients	Quantity
Beetroot	147 g
Soya Milk Unsweetened	7 ml
Almond Milk Unsweetened	150 ml
Coconut Oil	12 ml

Method

- Chop 147g beetroot into small pieces.
- Blend with 7ml unsweetened soya milk and 150 ml almond milk.
- Add 12ml coconut oil.
- Blend until smooth and creamy.
- Serve it.

Recipe by – Soma Basu

MILK

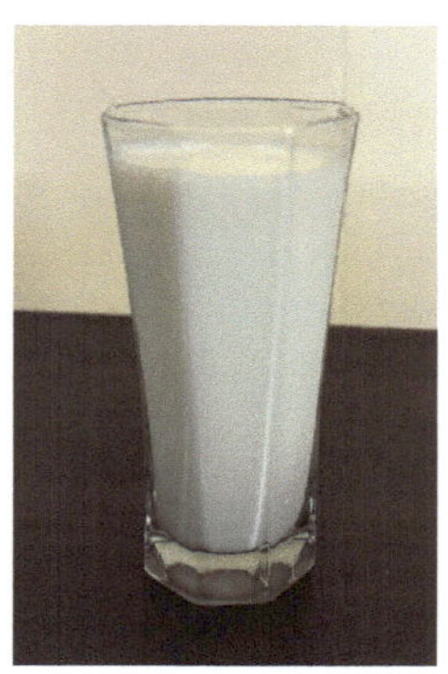
187 ml

Nutritive Value

Nutrient	Value
Energy (kcal)	158.47
Carbohydrates (g)	9.11
Protein (g)	3.08
Fat (g)	12.19

List of Ingredients

Ingredients	Quantity
Full Cream Milk	186 ml
Coconut Oil	1 ml

Method

- Take 186ml Full Cream Milk.
- Add 1ml Coconut Oil.
- Stir or blend well until smooth and uniform.
- Serve warm or chilled as preferred.

Recipe by – Soma Basu

COCONUT MILK

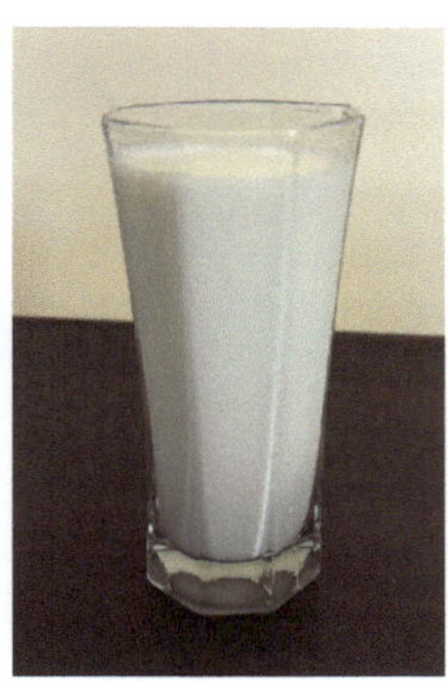

91 ml

Nutritive Value

Nutrient	Value
Energy (kcal)	158.47
Carbohydrates (g)	9.11
Protein (g)	3.08
Fat (g)	12.19

List of Ingredients

Ingredients	Quantity
Coconut Milk	77 ml
Soya Milk Unsweetened	14 ml

Method

- Mix 77ml coconut milk with 14ml Soya Milk (Unsweetened).
- Stir or blend well until smooth and uniform.
- Serve warm or chilled as preferred.

Recipe by – Soma Basu

BOILED EGG AND VEGETABLE

Nutritive Value

Nutrient	Value
Energy (kcal)	158.47
Carbohydrates (g)	9.11
Protein (g)	3.08
Fat (g)	12.19

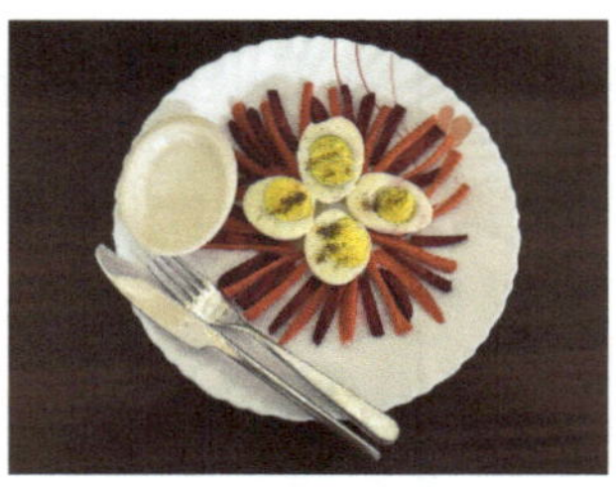

185 g

List of Ingredients

Ingredients	Quantity
Egg	11 g
Carrot	82 g
Beetroot	82 g
Coconut Oil	10 ml

Method

- Boil 11g egg, 82g carrot, and 82g beetroot until cooked.
- Chop all boiled ingredients into bite-sized pieces.
- Drizzle with 10ml coconut oil.
- Mix well and serve warm.

Recipe by – Soma Basu

COCONUT FLOUR LADOO

Nutritive Value

Nutrient	Value
Energy (kcal)	158.47
Carbohydrates (g)	9.11
Protein (g)	3.08
Fat (g)	12.19

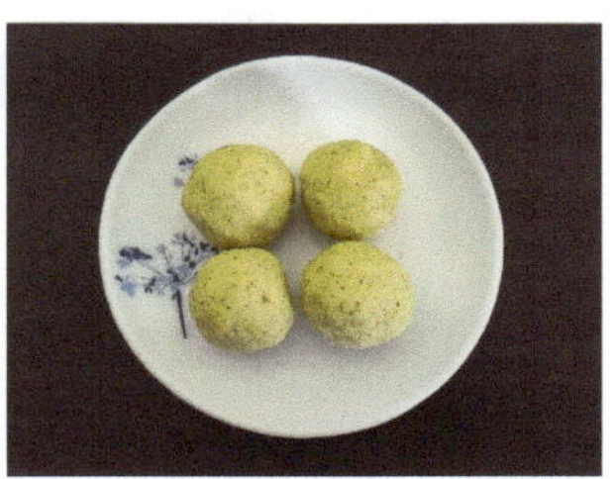

107 g

List of Ingredients

Ingredients	Quantity
Coconut Flour	16 g
Almond Milk Unsweetened	80 ml
Ghee	11 g

Method

- Heat 11g ghee in a pan.
- Add 16g coconut flour; roast on low flame until aromatic (2–3 mins).
- Pour in 80ml Almond Milk (Unsweetened); mix well to form a soft dough.
- Cool slightly, then shape into small ladoos.
- Serve or store in an airtight container.

Recipe by – Soma Basu

ALMOND FLOUR UPMA

Nutritive Value

Nutrient	Value
Energy (kcal)	158.47
Carbohydrates (g)	9.11
Protein (g)	3.08
Fat (g)	12.19

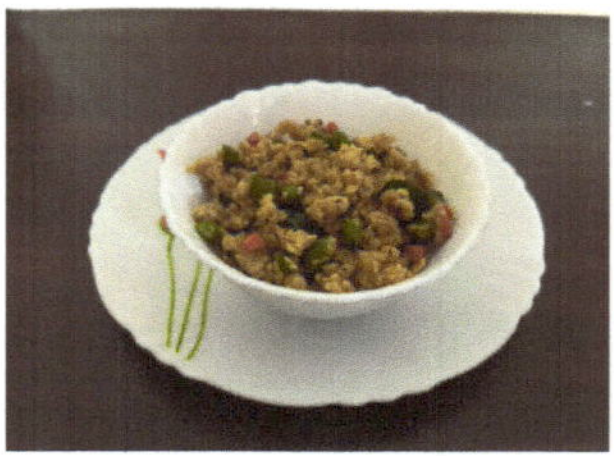

164 g

List of Ingredients

Ingredients	Quantity
Almond Flour	71 g
Carrot	81 g
Beans	10 g
Coconut Oil	2 ml

Method

- Heat 2ml coconut oil in a pan.
- Sauté 81g chopped carrots and 10g chopped beans until slightly soft.
- Add 71g almond flour and roast for 1–2 mins on low flame.
- Sprinkle a little water for moisture; cook until combined.
- Serve warm.

Recipe by – Soma Basu

ALMOND FLOUR PORRIDGE

Nutritive Value

Nutrient	Value
Energy (kcal)	158.47
Carbohydrates (g)	9.11
Protein (g)	3.08
Fat (g)	12.19

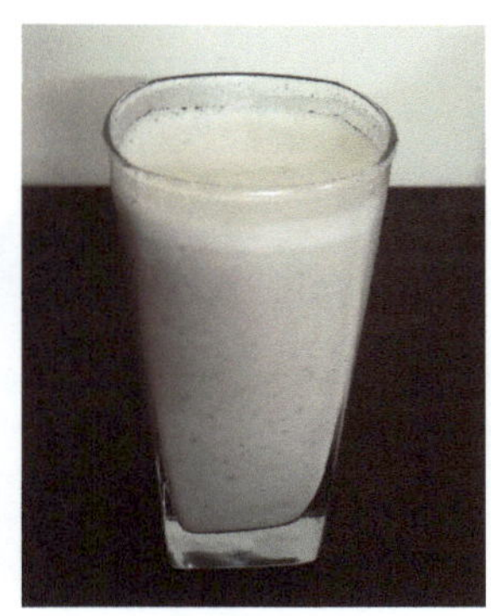

209 ml

List of Ingredients

Ingredients	Quantity
Almond Flour	71 g
Almond Milk Unsweetened	100 ml
Coconut Milk	38 ml

Method

- Heat 100ml Almond Milk (Unsweetened) and 38ml Coconut milk in a pan.
- Add 71g Almond Flour, stir to avoid lumps.
- Simmer on low heat for 3–4 mins until thick.
- Serve warm.

Recipe by – Soma Basu

ALMOND FLOUR HALWA

Nutritive Value

Nutrient	Value
Energy (kcal)	158.47
Carbohydrates (g)	9.11
Protein (g)	3.08
Fat (g)	12.19

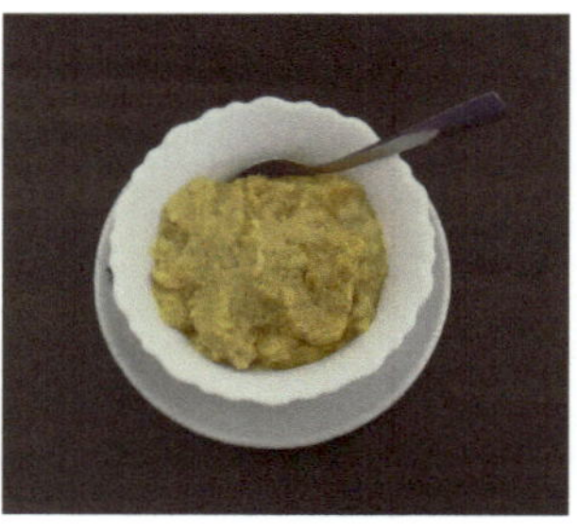

209 g

List of Ingredients

Ingredients	Quantity
Almond Flour	71 g
Coconut Milk	38 ml
Almond Milk Unsweetened	100 ml

Method

- Take 71g almond flour in pan; roast on low flame till aromatic.
- Pour in 100ml Almond Milk (Unsweetened) and 38ml Coconut Milk to it; stir continuously.
- Cook till the mixture thickens to halwa consistency.
- Serve warm.

Recipe by – Soma Basu

ALMOND FLOUR LADOO

Nutritive Value

Nutrient	Value
Energy (kcal)	158.47
Carbohydrates (g)	9.11
Protein (g)	3.08
Fat (g)	12.19

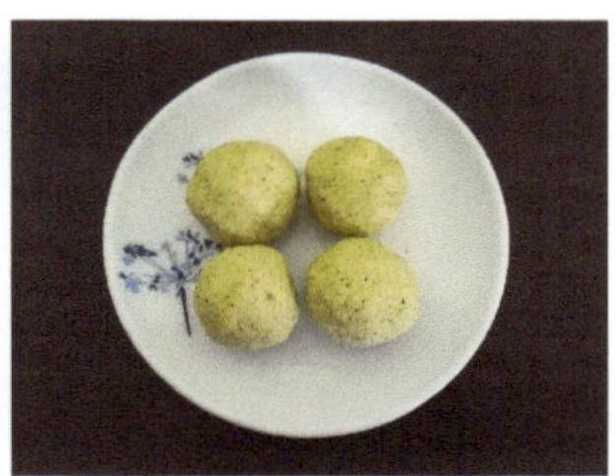

209 g

List of Ingredients

Ingredients	Quantity
Almond Flour	**71 g**
Almond Milk Unsweetened	**100 ml**
Coconut Milk	**38 ml**

Method

- Take 71g almond flour; roast on low flame until aromatic (2–3 mins).
- Pour in 100ml Almond Milk (Unsweetened) and 38ml Coconut Milk to it; mix well to form a soft dough.
- Cool slightly, then shape into small ladoos.
- Serve or store in an airtight container.

Recipe by – Soma Basu

ALMOND FLOUR DOSA + COCONUT CHUTNEY

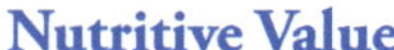

Nutritive Value

Nutrient	Value
Energy (kcal)	338.23
Carbohydrates (g)	9.11
Protein (g)	8.42
Fat (g)	29.79

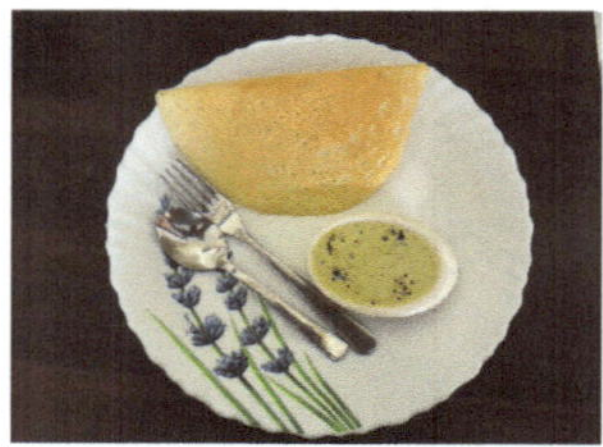

143 g

List of Ingredients

Ingredients	Quantity
Almond Flour	71 g
Coconut (for making chutney)	72 g

Method

- For dosa mix 71g Almond Flour with water to form a smooth, pourable batter.
- Add salt to taste.
- Heat non-stick pan, pour batter, and spread thin.
- Cook until golden on both sides.
- For chutney blend 72g Coconut with a little water, salt, and optional green chili.
- Serve dosa hot with coconut chutney.

Recipe by – Soma Basu

ALMOND FLOUR CHAPATI + EGG CURRY

Nutritive Value

Nutrient	Value
Energy (kcal)	184.58
Carbohydrates (g)	4.54
Protein (g)	7.54
Fat (g)	15.14

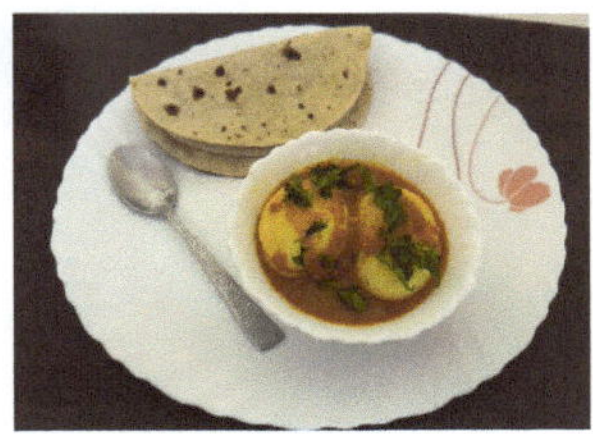

98 g

List of Ingredients

Ingredients	Quantity
Almond Flour	71 g
Egg (for making egg curry)	25 g
Coconut Oil	2 ml

Method

- For chapati mix 71g almond flour with a pinch of salt and warm water to form dough, roll gently into chapati shape.
- Cook on a hot pan using 1ml coconut oil (half of total oil).
- For egg curry boil 25g egg, peel and slice.
- Sauté mild spices (optional) in 1ml coconut oil.
- Add sliced egg, cook briefly.
- Serve with almond chapati.

Recipe by – Soma Basu

ALMOND FLOUR CHAPATI + CHICKEN CURRY

Nutritive Value

Nutrient	Value
Energy (kcal)	261.43
Carbohydrates (g)	4.54
Protein (g)	9.63
Fat (g)	22.75

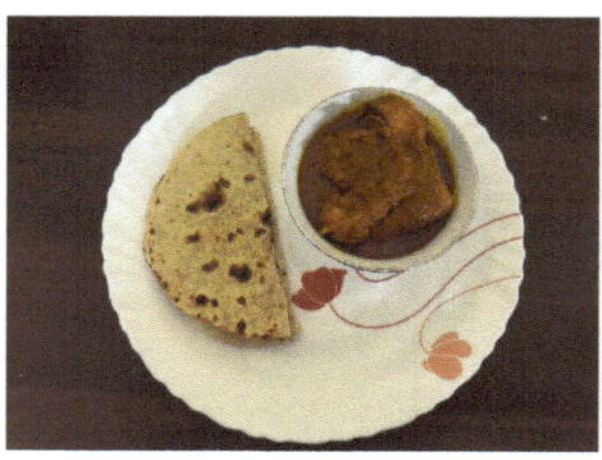

98 g

List of Ingredients

Ingredients	Quantity
Almond Flour	71 g
Chicken (for making chicken curry)	25 g
Coconut Oil	2 ml

Method

- For chapati mix 71g almond flour with a pinch of salt and warm water to form dough, roll gently into chapati shape.
- Cook on a hot pan until lightly golden on both sides
- For chicken curry heat 2ml coconut oil in a pan.
- Add 25g chicken. Sauté until cooked and slightly browned.
- Optional: Add spices (like turmeric, chili powder, salt) for flavor.
- Simmer with a splash of water to form a light curry.
- Serve hot chapati with chicken curry.

Recipe by – Soma Basu

ALMOND FLOUR CHAPATI + BEANS

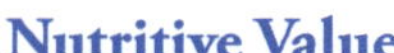

Nutrient	Value
Energy (kcal)	165.79
Carbohydrates (g)	6.68
Protein (g)	6.17
Fat (g)	12.71

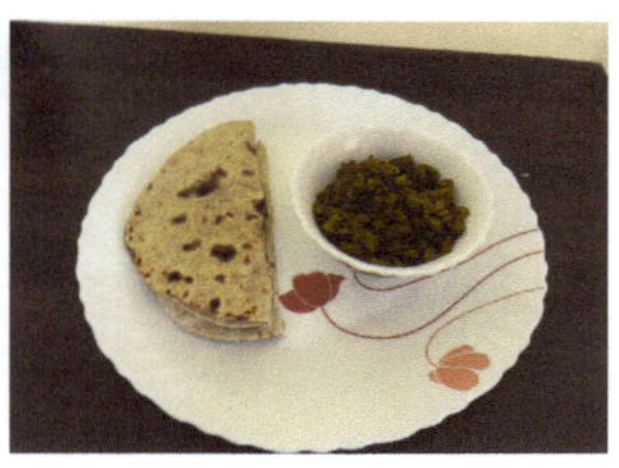

155 g

List of Ingredients

Ingredients	Quantity
Almond Flour	71 g
Beans	80 g
Coconut Oil	4 ml

Method

- For chapati mix 71g almond flour with a pinch of salt and warm water to form dough, roll gently into chapati shape.
- Cook on a hot pan until lightly golden on both sides
- For beans sabji chop 80g beans.
- Sauté in 4ml coconut oil until tender.
- Add salt and spices as desired (e.g., turmeric, cumin).
- Serve hot with almond chapatis.

Recipe by – Soma Basu

SAUTED VEGETABLES

Nutritive Value

Nutrient	Value
Energy (kcal)	208.27
Carbohydrates (g)	9.11
Protein (g)	6.53
Fat (g)	16.19

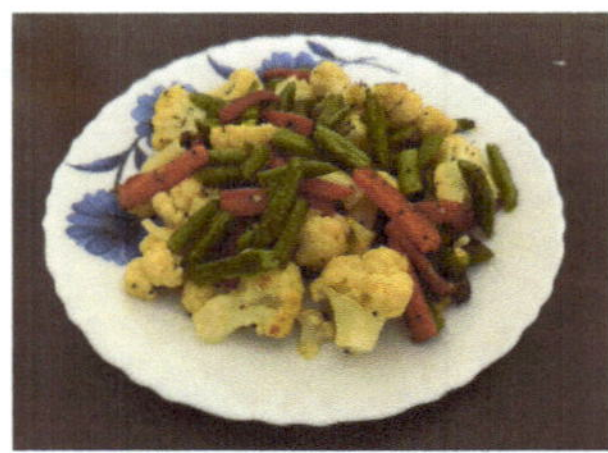

332 g

List of Ingredients

Ingredients	Quantity
Cauliflower	149 g
Carrot	55 g
Beans	113 g
Coconut Oil	15 ml

Method

- Chop 149g cauliflower, 55g carrot, and 113g beans into bite-sized pieces.
- Heat 15ml coconut oil in a pan.
- Add all veggies and sauté on medium heat.
- Cook for 5–7 mins until tender yet crisp.
- Season with salt and pepper (optional).
- Serve hot.

Recipe by – Soma Basu

ALMOND FLOUR POORI + SOYA CHUNKS

Nutritive Value

Nutrient	Value
Energy (kcal)	232.94
Carbohydrates (g)	3.84
Protein (g)	13.94
Fat (g)	17.98

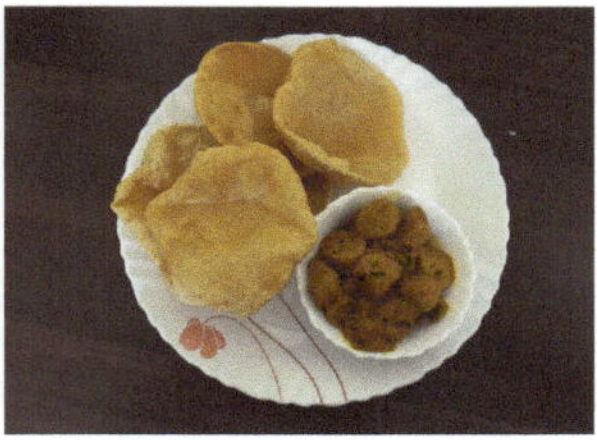

89 g

List of Ingredients

Ingredients	Quantity
Almond Flour	60 g
Soya Chunks	20 g
Coconut Oil	9 ml

Method

- For Almond Flour Poori in a bowl, mix 60 g almond flour with a pinch of salt. Add warm water little by little, knead into a soft dough roll small balls into flat pooris.
- Heat coconut oil (4.5 ml) in a pan, shallow fry pooris until golden.
- For Soya Chunk side dish boil 20 g soya chunks in water until soft, squeeze out excess water.
- Heat coconut oil (4.5 ml) in a pan.

Recipe by – Soma Basu

- Add spices (like turmeric, cumin, salt, chili powder). Sauté soya chunks until golden and slightly crispy.
- Serve hot Almond flour pooris with spicy soya chunk side dish.

PANEER STUFFED CAPSICUM

Nutritive Value

Nutrient	Value
Energy (kcal)	266
Protein (g)	11.8
Carbohydrate (g)	7
Fat (g)	20.2

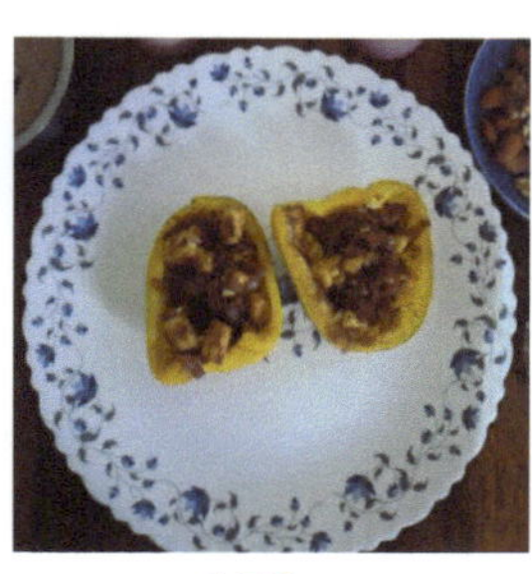

198 g

List Of Ingredients

Ingredients	Quantity
Medium capsicums (bell peppers)	100g
Paneer (crumbled)	60g
Onion (finely chopped)	15g
Tomato (finely chopped or pureed)	15g
Coriander leaves	chopped, for garnish
Oil or ghee	5ml (for sautéing and brushing)
Butter	3ml

Method

- Heat oil in a pan, sauté onion, ginger-garlic paste, tomato, and spices until soft.
- Add crumbled paneer, mix well, and cook for 2–3 minutes to make the stuffing.

Recipe by – Nishali A.M.

- Cut and deseed capsicums, stuff them with the paneer filling, and brush lightly with butter.
- Bake at 180°C for 15–20 minutes or cook covered on a pan until capsicums are tender.

Recipe by – Nishali A.M.

ORANGE MILKSHAKE

Nutritive Value

Nutrient	Value
Energy (kcal)	132
Protein (g)	0.8
Carbohydrate (g)	8.4
Fat (g)	9.55

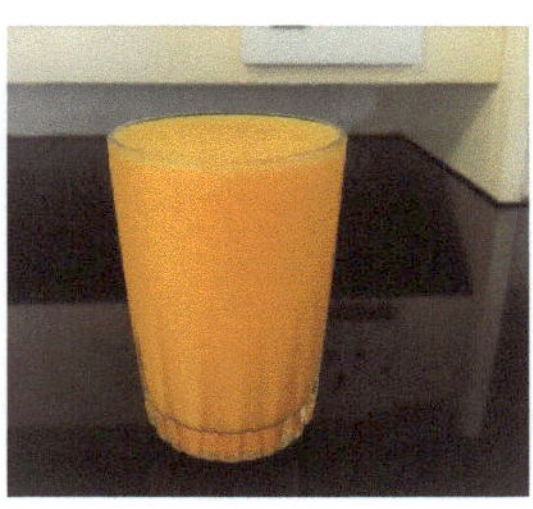

100 ml

List of Ingredients

Ingredients	Quantity
Fresh orange	40 g
Unsweetened almond milk	40 ml
Coconut oil	8.5ml

Method

- Extract fresh orange juice and strain to remove seeds/ pulp.
- In a blender, combine orange juice, chilled almond milk and coconut oil.
- Blend for a few seconds until smooth and frothy.
- Pour into a glass and serve immediately – enjoy fresh!

Recipe by – Nishali A.M.

MUSKMELON MILKSHAKE

Nutritive Value

Nutrient	Value
Energy (kcal)	65
Protein (g)	0.7
Carbohydrate (g)	4.3
Fat (g)	5

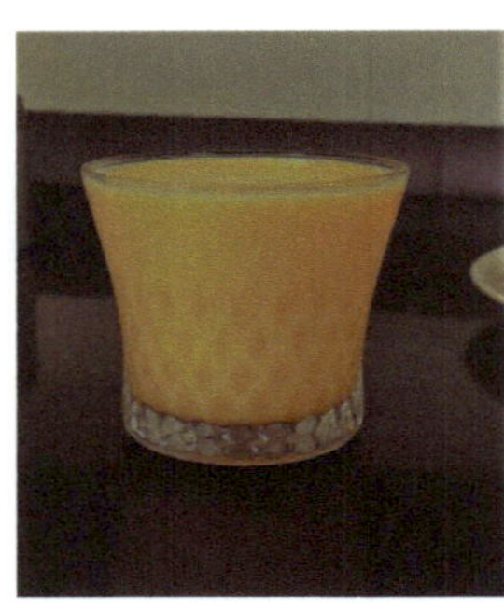

100 ml

List of Ingredients

Ingredients	Quantity
Chopped muskmelon	40 g
Chilled milk	30ml
Coconut oil	3.5ml
Cardamom powder	1g (optional, for flavor)

Method

- Blend muskmelon, milk, and cardamom powder until smooth.
- Add ice cubes and blend again for a chilled, frothy shake.
- Pour into a small glass and serve immediately.

Recipe by – Nishali A.M.

2:1 RATIO KETO RECIPES

APPLE MILKSHAKE

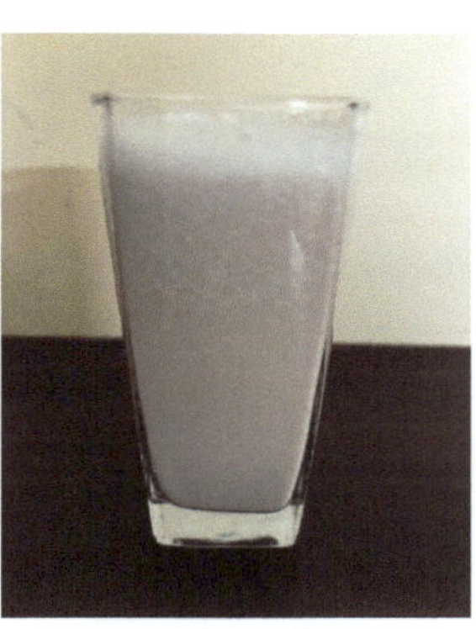
141 ml

Nutritive Value

Nutrient	Value
Energy (kcal)	158.49
Carbohydrates (g)	4.12
Protein (g)	3.08
Fat (g)	14.41

List of Ingredients

Ingredients	Quantity
Apple	32 g
Soya Milk Unsweetened	96 ml
Coconut Oil	13 ml

Method

- Chop 32g apple into small pieces.
- Blend with 96ml unsweetened soya milk.
- Add 13ml coconut oil.
- Blend until smooth and creamy.
- Serve it.

Recipe by – Soma Basu

BANANA MILKSHAKE

Nutritive Value

Nutrient	Value
Energy (kcal)	158.49
Carbohydrates (g)	4.12
Protein (g)	3.08
Fat (g)	14.41

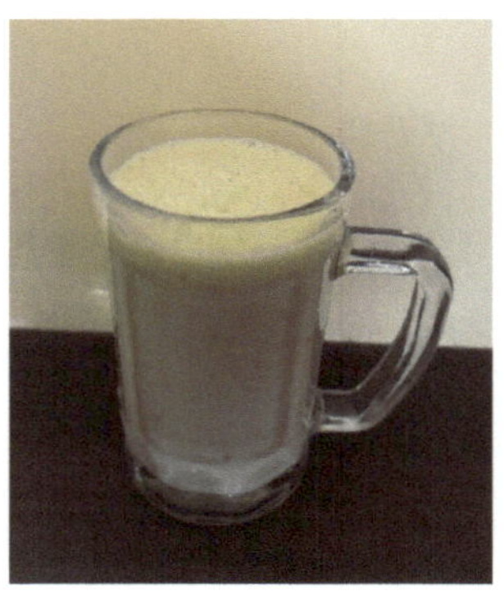

120 ml

List of Ingredients

Ingredients	Quantity
Banana	18 g
Soya Milk Unsweetened	89 ml
Coconut Oil	13 ml

Method

- Chop 18g banana into small pieces.
- Blend with 89ml unsweetened soya milk.
- Add 13ml coconut oil.
- Blend until smooth and creamy.
- Serve it.

Recipe by – Soma Basu

SAPOTA MILKSHAKE

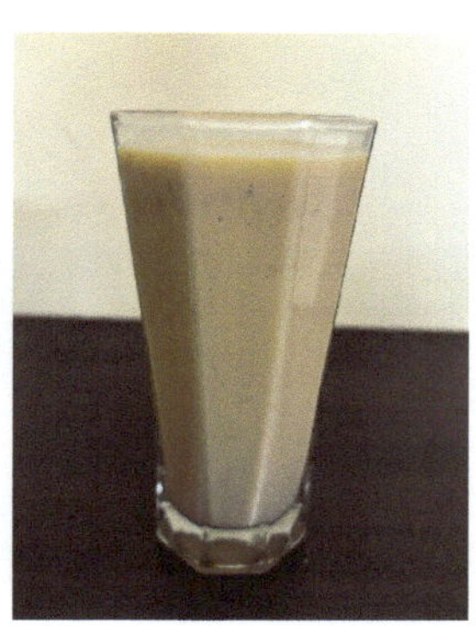

131 ml

Nutritive Value

Nutrient	Value
Energy (kcal)	158.49
Carbohydrates (g)	4.12
Protein (g)	3.08
Fat (g)	14.41

List of Ingredients

Ingredients	Quantity
Sapota	30 g
Soya Milk Unsweetened	88 ml
Coconut Oil	13 ml

Method

- Chop 30g sapota into small pieces.
- Blend with 88ml unsweetened soya milk.
- Add 13ml coconut oil.
- Blend until smooth and creamy.
- Serve it.

Recipe by – Soma Basu

POMEGRANATE MILKSHAKE

Nutritive Value

Nutrient	Value
Energy (kcal)	158.49
Carbohydrates (g)	4.12
Protein (g)	3.08
Fat (g)	14.41

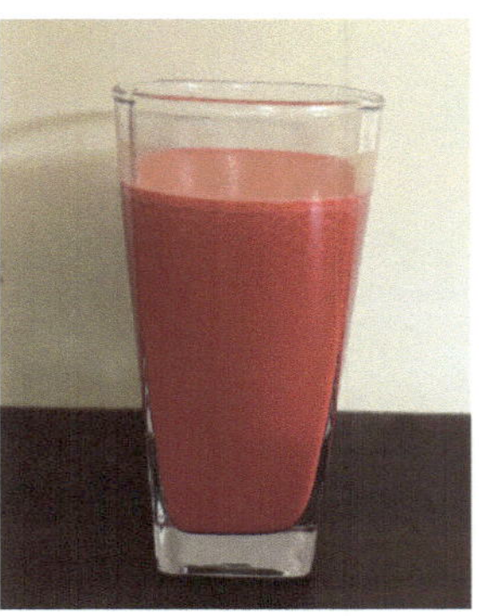

130 ml

List of Ingredients

Ingredients	Quantity
Pomegranate	36 g
Soya Milk Unsweetened	81 ml
Coconut Oil	13 ml

Method

- Chop 36g pomegranate into small pieces.
- Blend with 81ml unsweetened soya milk.
- Add 13ml coconut oil.
- Blend until smooth and creamy.
- Serve it.

Recipe by – Soma Basu

STRAWBERRY MILKSHAKE

Nutritive Value

Nutrient	Value
Energy (kcal)	158.49
Carbohydrates (g)	4.12
Protein (g)	3.08
Fat (g)	14.41

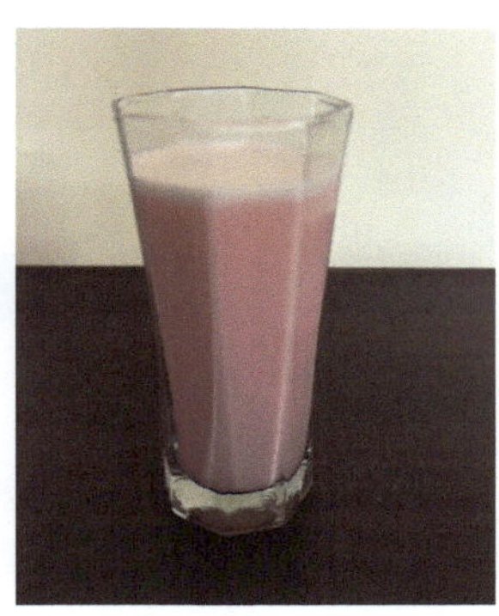

230 ml

List of Ingredients

Ingredients	Quantity
Strawberry	121 g
Soya Milk Unsweetened	94 ml
Coconut Oil	13 ml

Method

- Chop 121g strawberry into small pieces.
- Blend with 94ml unsweetened soya milk.
- Add 13ml coconut oil.
- Blend until smooth and creamy.
- Serve it.

Recipe by – Soma Basu

CARROT MILKSHAKE

Nutritive Value

Nutrient	Value
Energy (kcal)	158.49
Carbohydrates (g)	4.12
Protein (g)	3.08
Fat (g)	14.41

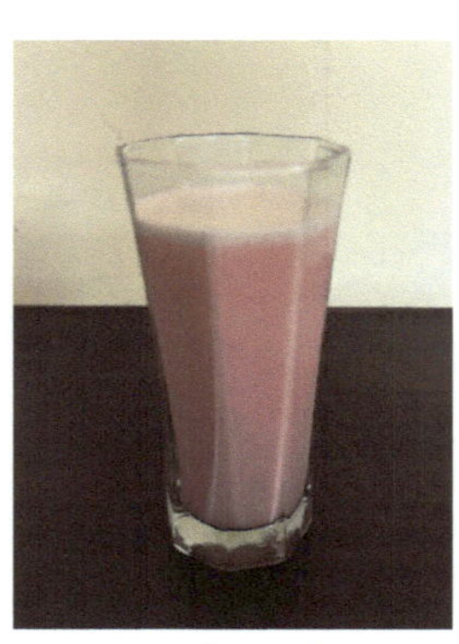

261 ml

List of Ingredients

Ingredients	Quantity
Carrot	74 g
Soya Milk Unsweetened	74 ml
Almond Milk Unsweetened	100 ml
Coconut Oil	13 ml

Method

- Chop 74g carrot into small pieces.
- Blend with 74ml unsweetened soya milk and 100 ml almond milk.
- Add 13ml coconut oil.
- Blend until smooth and creamy.
- Serve it.

Recipe by – Soma Basu

BEETROOT MILKSHAKE

Nutritive Value

Nutrient	Value
Energy (kcal)	158.49
Carbohydrates (g)	4.12
Protein (g)	3.08
Fat (g)	14.41

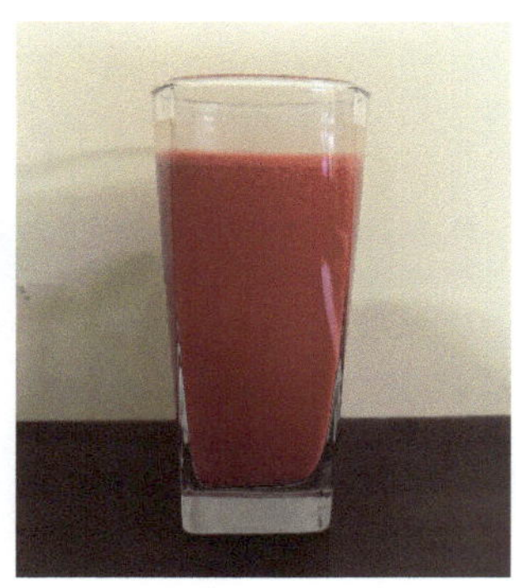

235 ml

List of Ingredients

Ingredients	Quantity
Beetroot	67 g
Soya Milk Unsweetened	55 ml
Almond Milk Unsweetened	100 ml
Coconut Oil	13 ml

Method

- Chop 67g beetroot into small pieces.
- Blend with 55ml unsweetened soya milk and 100 ml almond milk.
- Add 13ml coconut oil.
- Blend until smooth and creamy.
- Serve it.

Recipe by – Soma Basu

MILK MIX

Nutritive Value

Nutrient	Value
Energy (kcal)	158.49
Carbohydrates (g)	4.12
Protein (g)	3.08
Fat (g)	14.41

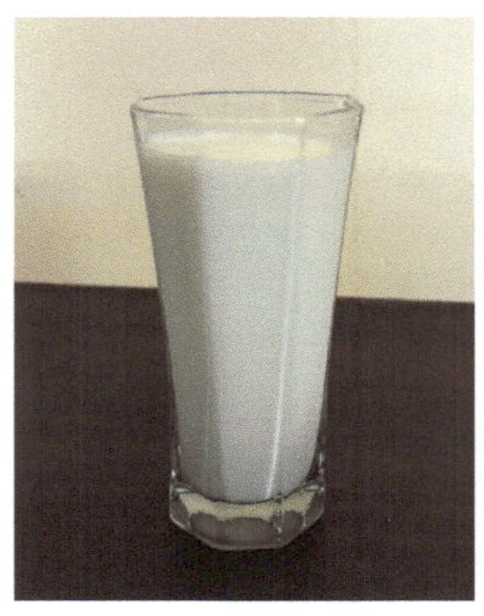

111 ml

List of Ingredients

Ingredients	Quantity
Full Cream Milk	84 ml
Soya Milk Unsweetened	18 ml
Coconut Oil	9 ml

Method

- Mix 84ml Full Cream Milk with 18ml Soya Milk (Unsweetened).
- Add 9ml Coconut Oil.
- Stir or blend well until smooth and uniform.
- Serve warm or chilled as preferred.

Recipe by – Soma Basu

COCONUT MILK

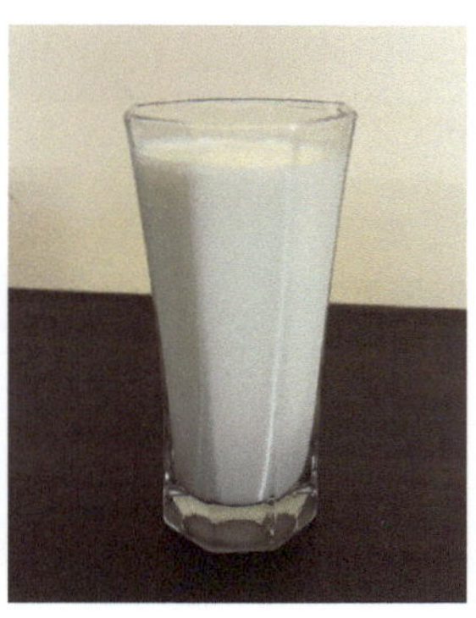

109 ml

Nutritive Value

Nutrient	Value
Energy (kcal)	158.49
Carbohydrates (g)	4.12
Protein (g)	3.08
Fat (g)	14.41

List of Ingredients

Ingredients	Quantity
Coconut Milk	35 ml
Soya Milk Unsweetened	59 ml
Coconut Oil	15 ml

Method

- Mix 35ml coconut milk with 59ml Soya Milk (Unsweetened).
- Add 15ml Coconut Oil.
- Stir or blend well until smooth and uniform.
- Serve warm or chilled as preferred.

Recipe by – Soma Basu

BOILED EGG AND VEGETABLE

Nutritive Value

Nutrient	Value
Energy (kcal)	158.49
Carbohydrates (g)	4.12
Protein (g)	3.08
Fat (g)	14.41

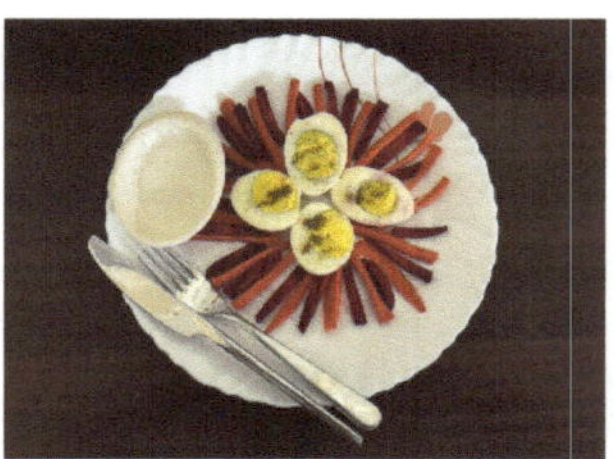

104 g

List of Ingredients

Ingredients	Quantity
Egg	18 g
Carrot	37 g
Beetroot	37 g
Coconut Oil	12 ml

Method

- Boil 18g egg, 37g carrot, and 37g beetroot until cooked.
- Chop all boiled ingredients into bite-sized pieces.
- Drizzle with 12ml coconut oil.
- Mix well and serve warm.

Recipe by – Soma Basu

ALMOND FLOUR UPMA

Nutritive Value

Nutrient	Value
Energy (kcal)	158.49
Carbohydrates (g)	4.12
Protein (g)	3.08
Fat (g)	14.41

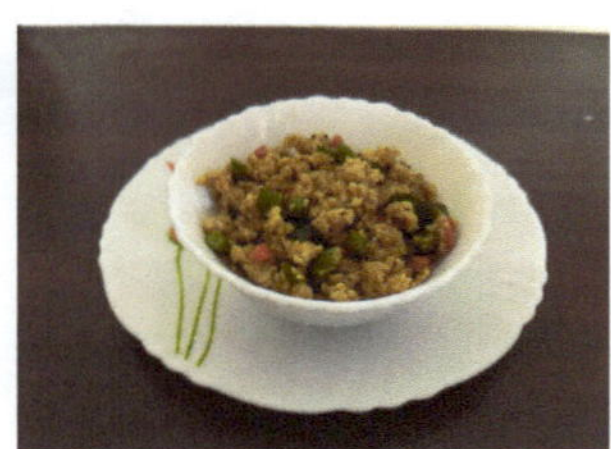

79 g

List of Ingredients

Ingredients	Quantity
Almond Flour	64 g
Carrot	5 g
Beans	5 g
Coconut Oil	5 ml

Method

- Heat 5ml coconut oil in a pan.
- Sauté 5g chopped carrots and 5g chopped beans until slightly soft.
- Add 64g almond flour and roast for 1–2 mins on low flame.
- Sprinkle a little water for moisture; cook until combined.
- Serve warm.

Recipe by – Soma Basu

ALMOND FLOUR HALWA

Nutritive Value

Nutrient	Value
Energy (kcal)	158.49
Carbohydrates (g)	4.12
Protein (g)	3.08
Fat (g)	14.41

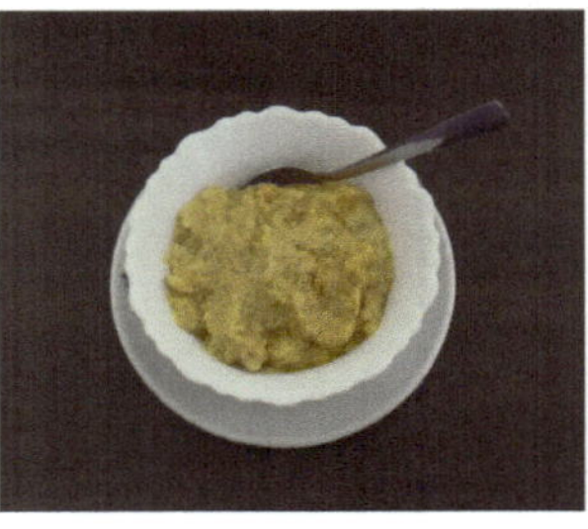

169 g

List of Ingredients

Ingredients	Quantity
Almond Flour	64 g
Almond Milk Unsweetened	100 ml
Ghee	5 g

Method

- Heat 5g ghee in a pan.
- Add 64g almond flour; roast on low flame till aromatic.
- Pour in 100ml Almond Milk (Unsweetened); stir continuously.
- Cook till the mixture thickens to halwa consistency.
- Serve warm.

Recipe by – Soma Basu

COCONUT FLOUR LADOO

Nutritive Value

Nutrient	Value
Energy (kcal)	158.49
Carbohydrates (g)	4.12
Protein (g)	3.08
Fat (g)	14.41

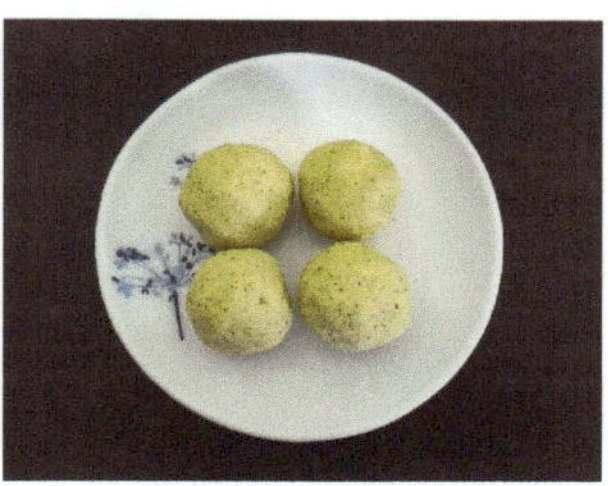

68 g

List of Ingredients

Ingredients	Quantity
Coconut Flour	7 g
Soya Milk Unsweetened	48 ml
Ghee	13 g

Method

- Heat 13g ghee in a pan.
- Add 7g coconut flour; roast on low flame until aromatic (2–3 mins).
- Pour in 48ml Soya Milk (Unsweetened); mix well to form a soft dough.
- Cool slightly, then shape into small ladoos.
- Serve or store in an airtight container.

Recipe by – Soma Basu

ALMOND FLOUR LADOO

Nutritive Value

Nutrient	Value
Energy (kcal)	158.49
Carbohydrates (g)	4.12
Protein (g)	3.08
Fat (g)	14.41

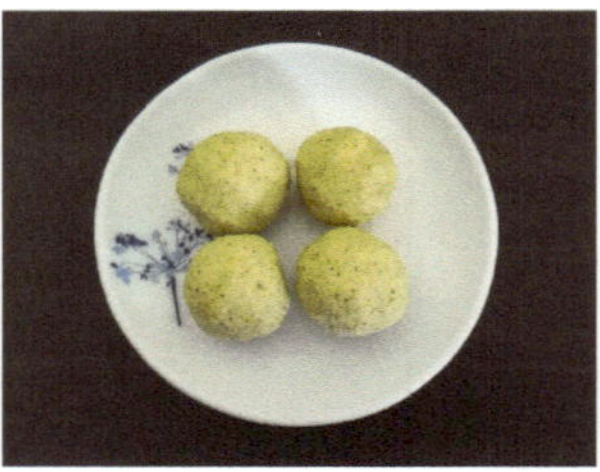

169 g

List of Ingredients

Ingredients	Quantity
Almond Flour	64 g
Almond Milk Unsweetened	100 ml
Ghee	5 g

Method

- Heat 5g ghee in a pan.
- Add 64g almond flour; roast on low flame until aromatic (2–3 mins).
- Pour in 100ml Almond Milk (Unsweetened); mix well to form a soft dough.
- Cool slightly, then shape into small ladoos.
- Serve or store in an airtight container.

Recipe by – Soma Basu

ALMOND FLOUR PORRIDGE

Nutritive Value

Nutrient	Value
Energy (kcal)	158.49
Carbohydrates (g)	4.12
Protein (g)	3.08
Fat (g)	14.41

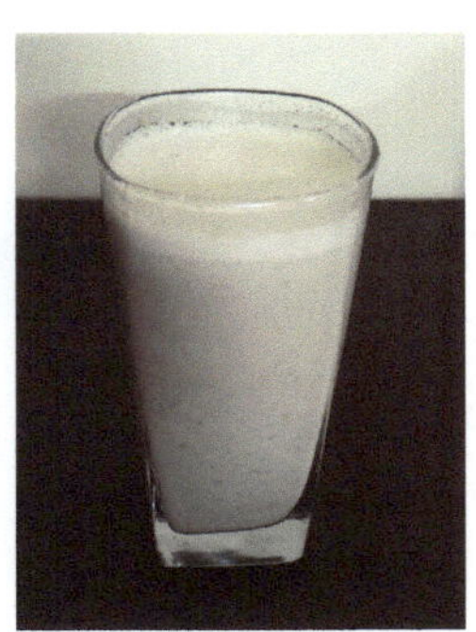

219 ml

List of Ingredients

Ingredients	Quantity
Almond Flour	64 g
Almond Milk Unsweetened	150 ml
Coconut Oil	5 ml

Method

- Heat 150ml Almond Milk (Unsweetened) in a pan.
- Add 64g Almond Flour, stir to avoid lumps.
- Simmer on low heat for 3–4 mins until thick.
- Mix in 5ml Coconut Oil before serving.
- Serve warm.

Recipe by – Soma Basu

ALMOND FLOUR DOSA + COCONUT CHUTNEY

Nutritive Value

Nutrient	Value
Energy (kcal)	158.49
Carbohydrates (g)	4.12
Protein (g)	3.08
Fat (g)	14.41

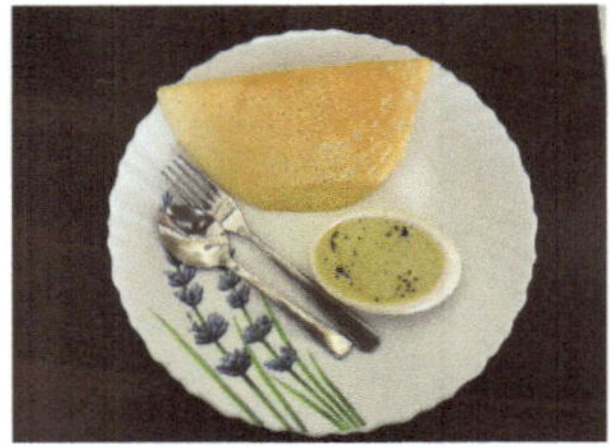

65 g

List of Ingredients

Ingredients	Quantity
Almond Flour	32 g
Coconut (for making chutney)	33 g

Method

- For dosa mix 32g Almond Flour with water to form a smooth, pourable batter.
- Add salt to taste.
- Heat non-stick pan, pour batter, and spread thin.
- Cook until golden on both sides.
- For chutney blend 33g Coconut with a little water, salt, and optional green chili.
- Serve dosa hot with coconut chutney.

Recipe by – Soma Basu

ALMOND FLOUR CHAPATI + EGG CURRY

Nutritive Value

Nutrient	Value
Energy (kcal)	230.2
Carbohydrates (g)	4.12
Protein (g)	6.18
Fat (g)	21

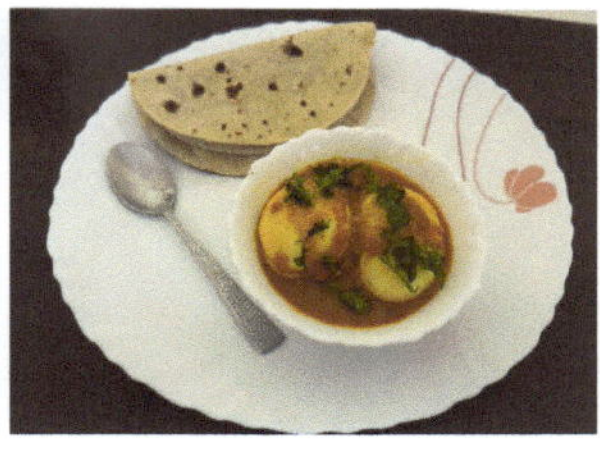

89 g

List of Ingredients

Ingredients	Quantity
Almond Flour	64 g
Egg (for making egg curry)	18 g
Coconut Oil	7 ml

Method

- For chapati mix 64g almond flour with a pinch of salt and warm water to form dough, roll gently into chapati shape.
- Cook on a hot pan using 3.5ml coconut oil (half of total oil).
- For egg curry boil 18g egg, peel and slice.
- Sauté mild spices (optional) in 3.5ml coconut oil.
- Add sliced egg, cook briefly.
- Serve with almond chapati.

Recipe by – Soma Basu

ALMOND FLOUR CHAPATI + CHICKEN CURRY

Nutritive Value

Nutrient	Value
Energy (kcal)	274
Carbohydrates (g)	4.12
Protein (g)	8.13
Fat (g)	25

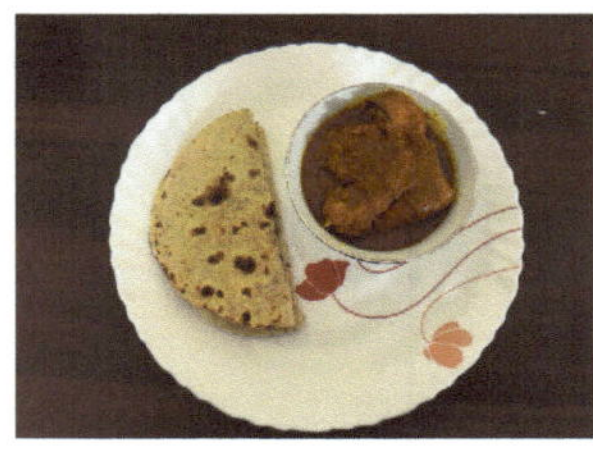

95 g

List of Ingredients

Ingredients	Quantity
Almond Flour	64 g
Chicken (for making chicken curry)	20 g
Coconut Oil	11 ml

Method

- For chapati mix 64g almond flour with a pinch of salt and warm water to form dough, roll gently into chapati shape.
- Cook on a hot pan until lightly golden on both sides
- For chicken curry heat 11ml coconut oil in a pan.
- Add 20g chicken. Sauté until cooked and slightly browned.

Recipe by – Soma Basu

- Optional: Add spices (like turmeric, chili powder, salt) for flavor.
- Simmer with a splash of water to form a light curry.
- Serve hot chapati with chicken curry.

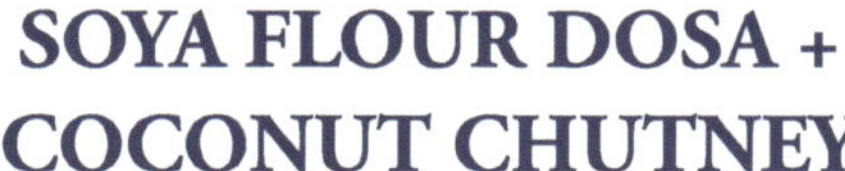

SOYA FLOUR DOSA + COCONUT CHUTNEY

Nutritive Value

Nutrient	Value
Energy (kcal)	321.07
Carbohydrates (g)	4.12
Protein (g)	9.42
Fat (g)	29.65

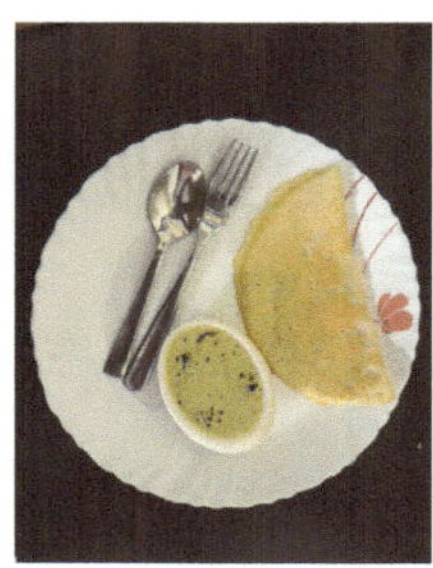

97 g

List of Ingredients

Ingredients	Quantity
Soya Flour	32 g
Coconut (for making chutney)	65 g

Method

- For dosa mix 32g Soya Flour with water to form a smooth, pourable batter.
- Add salt to taste.
- Heat non-stick pan, pour batter, and spread thin.
- Cook until golden on both sides.
- For chutney blend 65g Coconut with a little water, salt, and optional green chili.
- Serve dosa hot with coconut chutney.

Recipe by – Soma Basu

ALMOND FLOUR CHAPATI + BEANS

Nutritive Value

Nutrient	Value
Energy (kcal)	158.49
Carbohydrates (g)	4.12
Protein (g)	3.08
Fat (g)	14.41

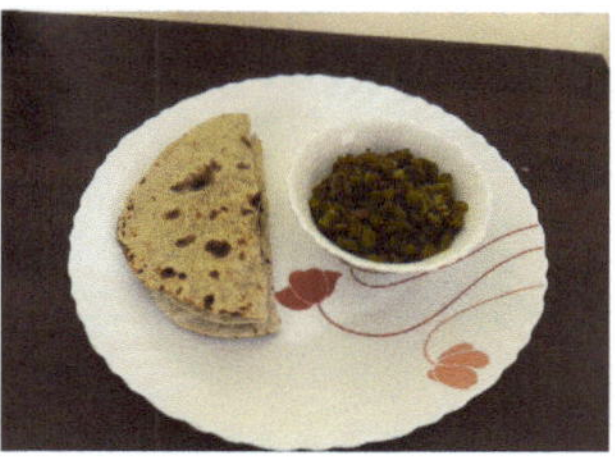

119 g

List of Ingredients

Ingredients	Quantity
Almond Flour	32 g
Beans	77 g
Coconut Oil	10 ml

Method

- For chapati mix 32g almond flour with a pinch of salt and warm water to form dough, roll gently into chapati shape.
- Cook on a hot pan until lightly golden on both sides
- For beans sabji chop 77g beans.
- Sauté in 10ml coconut oil until tender.
- Add salt and spices as desired (e.g., turmeric, cumin).
- Serve hot with almond chapatis.

Recipe by – Soma Basu

SAUTED VEGETABLES

Nutritive Value

Nutrient	Value
Energy (kcal)	158.49
Carbohydrates (g)	4.12
Protein (g)	3.08
Fat (g)	14.41

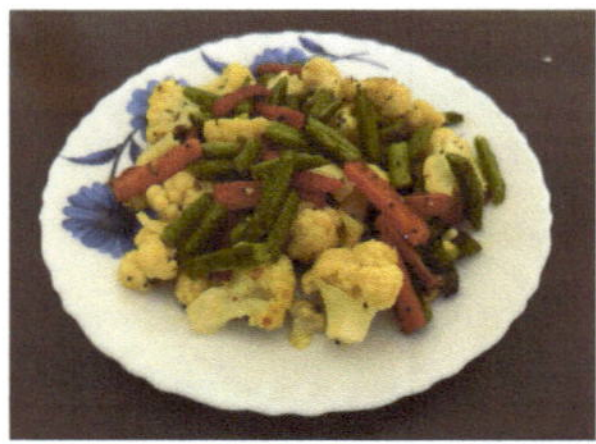

158 g

List of Ingredients

Ingredients	Quantity
Cauliflower	68 g
Carrot	25 g
Beans	51 g
Coconut Oil	14 ml

Method

- Chop 68g cauliflower, 25g carrot, and 51g beans into bite-sized pieces.
- Heat 14ml coconut oil in a pan.
- Add all veggies and sauté on medium heat.
- Cook for 5–7 mins until tender yet crisp.
- Season with salt and pepper (optional).
- Serve hot.

Recipe by – Soma Basu

ROASTED NUTS

Nutritive Value

Nutrient	Value
Energy (kcal)	241
Protein (g)	4.58
Carbohydrate (g)	4.5
Fat (g)	18.2

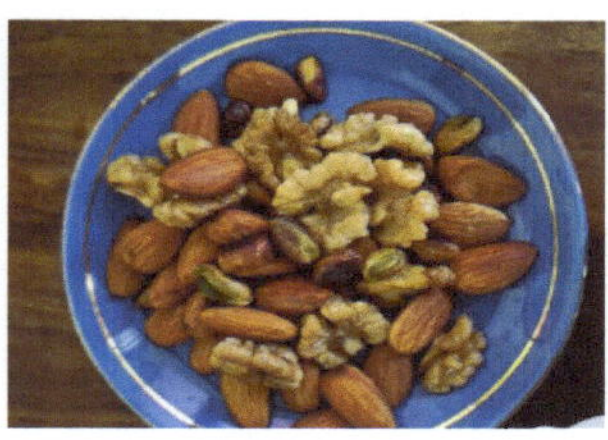

29 g

List of Ingredients

Ingredients	Quantity
Almonds	8g
Pistachio	8g
Walnuts	8g
Coconut Oil	5ml

Method

- Toss almonds, walnuts, and pistachios with coconut oil, salt, and spices of your choice.
- Roast at 170°C (340°F) for 12–15 minutes, stirring once, then cool and store.

Recipe by – Nishali A.M.

3:1 RATIO KETO RECIPES

DAHI SEEDS SALAD

Nutritive Value

Nutrient	Value
Energy (kcal)	283
Protein (g)	4.6
Fat (g)	26
Carbohydrate (g)	4

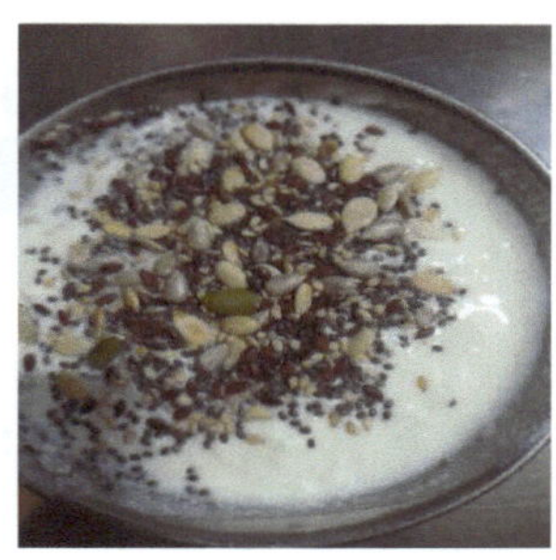

81 g

List of Ingredients

Ingredients	Quantity
Sunflower seed	3gm
Pumpkin seed	3gm
Chia seed	3gm
Flax seed	5 gm
Full fat Curd/ yogurt	50gm
Coconut oil	17ml

Method

- In a bowl, combine all seeds.
- Add curd and mix well.
- Drizzle in the coconut oil and stir until fully combined.
- Add salt if desired. Let it sit for 5–10 minutes for chia to swell a bit.
- Serve slightly chilled or at room temperature.

Recipe by – Trisha S

KETO PEANUT SALAD

Nutritive Value

Nutrient	Value
Energy (kcal)	340
Protein (g)	8
Fat (g)	30
Carbohydrate (g)	2

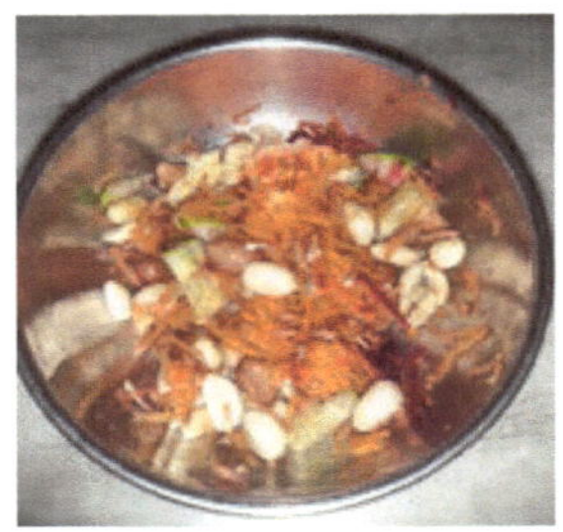

60 g

List of Ingredients

Ingredients	Quantity
Roasted peanuts	30gm
Onion	5gm
Tomato	5gm
capsicum	5gm
Walnuts	15gm
Salt, Black pepper, coriander, Lemon Juice	As per taste

Method

- In a bowl, combine chopped onion, tomato, and capsicum.
- Add roasted peanuts.
- Drizzle with coconut oil and mix gently.
- Season with salt, pepper, and lemon juice if using.
- Garnish with coriander leaves and serve fresh

Recipe by – Trisha S

DAHI PANEER KEBAB

Nutritive Value

Nutrient	Value
Energy (kcal)	336
Protein (g)	7.91
Carbohydrate (g)	5.67
Fat (g)	40.74

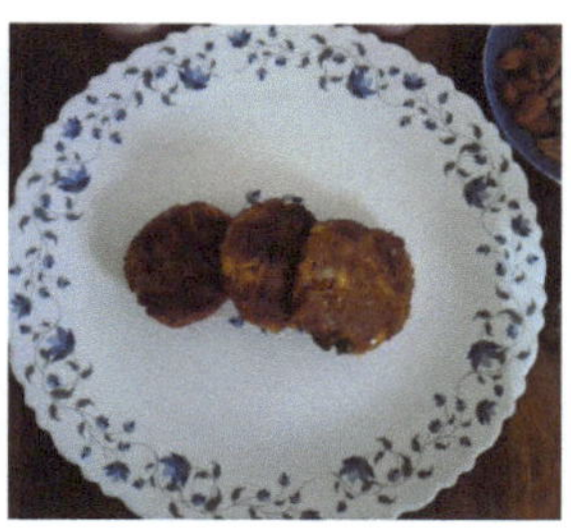

101 g

List of Ingredients

Ingredients	Quantity
Paneer (grated or crumbled)	30g
Thick curd (hung curd preferred)	13g
Onion (finely chopped)	15g
Green chili & ginger (finely chopped)	5g
Coriander leaves –	2g
Coconut Oil	26ml
Butter	10g

Methods

- Mix paneer, curd, besan, onion, chili, ginger, coriander, spices, butter and salt into a soft dough.
- Shape into small kebabs or patties (2–3 pieces, depending on size).

Recipe by – Trisha S

- Heat oil in a pan and shallow-fry on medium heat until golden on both sides.
- Serve hot with mint chutney or yogurt dip.

www.ingramcontent.com/pod-product-compliance
Ingram Content Group UK Ltd.
Pitfield, Milton Keynes, MK11 3LW, UK
UKHW060358300726

14090UKWH00001B/14

* 9 7 9 8 8 9 9 0 6 9 9 8 7 *